They've Had a Good Innings

CORNWALL COLLEGE
LEARNING CENTRE

They've Had a Good Innings: Can the NHS Cope with an Ageing Population?

John Grimley Evans
Stephen Pollard
Karol Sikora
Roger Williams

Introduction by
David G. Green
and
Benedict Irvine

Civitas: Institute for the Study of Civil Society
London

First published May 2003
Civitas
The Mezzanine, Elizabeth House
39 York Road, London SE1 7NQ
email: books@civitas.org.uk

ISBN 1-903 386-27 6

These essays began as papers given at a conference: 'Living Longer: Can the NHS Cope?', held in November 2002. We are grateful to Merck, Sharp and Dohme for generously contributing to the cost of the seminar.

Typeset by Civitas
in New Century Schoolbook

Printed in Great Britain by

Hartington Fine Arts Ltd
Lancing, Sussex

Contents

Authors

Stephen Pollard is a Senior Fellow at the Centre for the New Europe in Brussels, where he directs the health policy programme and edits www.cnehealth.org. He is currently writing a biography of David Blunkett, which will be published in spring 2005. He also writes and broadcasts on public policy and politics. His columns appear in many newspapers, and regularly in *The Times*, *Sunday Telegraph* and *Wall Street Journal Europe*. From 1998-2001 he was political columnist and chief leader writer for the *Daily Express*. Before that he was head of research at the Social Market Foundation, and from 1992-95 he was research director for the Fabian Society, the Labour Party's think tank. He is the author of numerous books including the best-selling *A Class Act: The myth of Britain's classless society* (with Andrew Adonis) Penguin, 1998. He became senior fellow at Civitas in 2001.

Karol Sikora is special adviser to HCA International in the creation of the London Cancer Group—the largest UK cancer network outside the NHS in HCA's six major London private hospitals. This includes the construction of a new international cancer centre for care, teaching and research in London at the Harley Street Clinic. He is also Global Clinical Expert to AstraZeneca, Oncology. He is Professor of Cancer Medicine and honorary Consultant Oncologist at Imperial College School of Medicine, Hammersmith Hospital, London where he was clinical director for 12 years. From 1997-99 he was chief of the WHO Cancer Programme based in Lyon, and from 1999-2001 Vice President, Global Clinical Research (Oncology) at Pharmacia Corporation.

He has published over 300 papers and written or edited 17 books including *Treatment of Cancer*—the standard British postgraduate textbook now in its fourth edition. He is on the editorial board of several journals and is the founding editor of *Gene Therapy and Cancer Strategy*. He is a former member of the UK Health Department's Expert Advisory Group on Cancer (the Calman-Hine Committee), the Committee on Safety of Medicines and remains an adviser to the WHO Cancer Programme.

Sir John Grimley Evans is Emeritus Professor of Clinical Geratology in the Nuffield Department of Clinical Medicine, University of Oxford, and Emeritus Fellow of Green College, Oxford. He studied natural sciences and clinical medicine at the Universities of Cambridge and Oxford. After postgraduate training and experience in clinical epidemiology at Oxford and the University of Michigan (USA), he carried out research work on migrant populations in the South West Pacific. From 1969 to 1971, he was lecturer in epidemiology at the London School of Hygiene and Tropical Medicine. Then, from 1971 to 1984 he worked as Consultant Physician in Geriatric and General Medicine and Professor of Medicine (Geriatrics) at the University of Newcastle upon Tyne. He was appointed Emeritus Professor of Clinical Geratology at Nuffield Department of Clinical Medicine, Oxford, in 1985. He is co-ordinating editor of *Clinicial Matters*, the journal of the Cochrane Dementia and Cognitive Improvement Group.

He has served as second vice-president of the Royal College of Physicians, member of Medical Research Council, chairman of MRC Health Services and Public Health Research Board. He was knighted in 1997 for his services to geriatric medicine in the UK.

Roger Williams' work in clinical liver disease and research has brought him a national and international reputation and has been marked by presidencies of both the British and European Associations for the Study of the Liver in 1983-85 and 1983 respectively. He has published over 2,500 papers, journals and books and has served on 22 editorial boards. The Liver Unit that he started at King's College Hospital in 1966 was recognised as an Institute of Liver Studies by King's College, London in 1990.

Professor Williams was honoured by election as Fellow of the Royal College of Surgeons in recognition of his contribution to the development of liver transplantation and has also been given the Fellowship of the Edinburgh College and that of the Royal College of Physicians of Australasia. In 1992 he was made a Fellow of King's College, London, and in that year was also awarded an Honorary Fellowship of the American College of Physicians. He was appointed a CBE in the Queen's Birthday Honours list of 1993, and the title of Professor of Hepatology was conferred by the University of London in May 1994.

From October 1996, Professor Williams continued his commitment to hepatology as Director of the Institute of Hepatology at University College London and Honorary Consultant Physician in Medicine at UCL Hospitals Trust. His aim is to make the Institute, which was established by the Foundation for Liver Research (formerly the Liver Research Trust), a centre of excellence in the UK and to forge links with other liver centres around the world in areas of work including virus induced liver disease, auto-immune liver disorders, gene therapy, novel therapeutic agents and bio-artificial liver support devices. In 2002 Professor Williams was appointed President of the British Liver Trust.

Foreword

For many years, we have been accustomed to thinking that the NHS will treat us from cradle to grave. But has this ever been a reality? Moreover, how will the ageing of the population and advances in medical technology affect the cost of health care in the future?

To explore these issues, Civitas set up a half-day, round-table conference with a panel of internationally recognised practitioners and opinion leaders. These essays were produced for that discussion and substantially modified as a result of the debate.

David G. Green

Introduction

David G. Green
Benedict Irvine

We all fear the prospect of becoming ill and dependent in old age and it is reassuring to feel that we can count on the National Health Service. But as more and more doctors speak out about gaps in NHS cover, can we be sure it will be there when we need it? Not only are there good reasons for worrying about the ability of the NHS to cope, there is now strong evidence of deliberate discrimination against the elderly. At the very time we need care most, it may be withheld because a doctor takes the view that we have 'had a good innings'.

The latest publication of the OECD's health data has again shown the poor quality of British healthcare compared with other countries.[1] The statistics show that victims of heart disease, stroke or breast cancer in Britain die early and unnecessarily compared with most other Western countries. Worse still, it seems that access to care is being limited according to age. In 2002, Roger Dobson, regular contributor to the *British Medical Journal*, reported on an international study that found the proportion of health spending on those aged 65+ in England and Wales was not keeping track with that in other countries.[2] Dr Alastair Gray and Meena Seshamani from the Health Economics Research Centre at Oxford University found:

> In contrast to the findings of previous studies, this analysis of health expenditure data has found that in England and Wales the high cost older groups did not have larger increases in their medical costs than the middle age groups. In fact...the oldest old had decreases in their real *per capita* costs, while other age groups experienced real cost increases.[3]

1

The same researchers noted that data from the OECD show that in developed countries *per capita* spending for those aged over 65 has increased at the same rate or faster than among those aged under 65. The UK bucks this trend.

Worse still, the NHS fails to provide health care for some elderly people even when the improvement in health status would be the same or greater than for younger people. A study in 1993 found that some coronary care units had upper age limits, even though there is no evidence that older people who have suffered acute heart attacks benefit less than younger people from specialist cardiological care. These examples of discrimination occur, argues Professor Grimley Evans of Oxford's Radcliffe Infirmary, because of 'poor science and woolly ethics'.[4]

A study of the NHS in Northern Ireland found that some doctors' judgements about which patients should be given priority for heart surgery were influenced by age, as well as other characteristics such as smoking and 'body mass'. In plain English, people who were fat, old or smoked were given lower priority.[5]

The frequency of use of medical interventions of recognised effectiveness can also be employed as an indicator of systematic discrimination. For example, two types of heart disease operations, coronary artery bypass grafting (CABG or 'cabbages' in medical slang) and percutaneous transluminal coronary angioplasty (PTCA), are considered effective treatments for relieving pain, preventing heart attacks and prolonging life.[6] PTCA has seen increases in prevalence in recent years but, according to a study by the OECD's Ageing Related Disease (ARD) Team, there is considerable variation between OECD countries.[7]

A Scottish study found that older patients who had been admitted to hospital because of a heart attack were afforded less extensive investigation (angiography) and fewer treatments, including CABGs, than younger patients. Angiography involves taking x-rays of arteries after the injection of a dye. It was provided for 38 per cent of the under 50s; 27 per cent of the 50-59 year olds; 14 per cent of the 60-69 year olds; but only three per cent of those aged 70 plus.[8]

There was a similar failure to carry out coronary artery bypass grafts. They were provided for ten per cent of the under 50s; 11 per cent of the 50-59 years olds; but only six per cent of the 60-69 year olds; and a mere one per cent of those aged 70 or more.[9] Yet, studies of patients in their 80s have found that, if operated on when the disease is still under control, they can tolerate surgery and enjoy a quality and quantity of life similar to that of others in their age group.[10]

The OECD ARD Team also compared stroke one-year case fatality in a number of centres in Europe and North America. Again the UK fatality rates are significantly worse for all age groups, but those for patients aged 75+ are particularly poor—approaching 57 per cent for men and 60 per cent for women, while rates in Denmark are c.30 per cent for men and c.25 per cent for women.[11]

Many elderly people are conscious that advancing age has led the NHS to treat them differently. In April 1999 a Gallup survey commissioned by Age Concern asked a random sample of adults aged over 50: 'Do you feel the NHS has ever dealt with you differently since you have been 50 or older?' Ten per cent of all respondents said 'yes'; eight per cent of those aged 50-64 said 'yes'; and 13 per cent of those aged 65 and over answered 'yes'.

If anything, they underestimated the extent of the discrimination. Breast cancer screening is offered every three years to women aged 50-64 in England and Wales. Despite the fact that the risk increases with age, most women over 65 must request a mammogram and, when they do so, there is evidence that obstacles are sometimes put in their way.[12] Several studies have found that screening 65-69 year olds produces the same 20-30 per cent reduction in mortality as in 50-64 year olds.[13] A study of women in the Netherlands found that regular mammographic screening of women over age 65 (and at least up to age 75) could reduce breast cancer deaths by about 45 per cent.[14]

Stephane Jacobzone *et al* at the OECD have also drawn attention to evidence that older women in the UK may not be receiving a regular mammogram. In Canada 65-70 per cent of women aged 50-60 reported receiving a mammogram in the preceding two years and this percentage fell to 44-49 for those 70 and over. But only 3.2 per cent of those 70+ in the UK reported having a mammogram in the past year compared to 40 per cent of those aged between 50 and 59 years.[15] In the face of this evidence of benefit to those over 64, in 2000 the National Screening Committee recommended that those aged 65-69, should also be invited for screening. This reform was duly announced in the *Cancer Plan*, and is to be implemented in England by 2004.[16] In 1998, a major US study, the Breast Cancer Detection Demonstration Project, found that five-year survival for women aged 60 or more was not very different from that for younger age groups. Death from breast cancer after five years occurred in 7.4 per cent of those aged under 50; in 8.5 per cent of those aged 50-59; and in 9.7 per cent of women aged 60 or more.[17]

But there are significant variations in cancer survival between countries, with the UK being below average. Four groups emerged when breast cancer survival was compared in the EUROCARE II Study. Switzerland and France were in the best performing group, Denmark, the Netherlands and Germany in the second group. Scotland and England (with Slovenia) were below average in a third group, while Slovakia, Poland and Estonia were in the worst performing group. While most countries presented a stable or increasing survival rate with increasing age of patients, England, Scotland, Slovakia, Poland and Estonia showed lower survival for the elderly.[18] Of eight countries for which data were collected by the OECD in 2002, England had the lowest five-year survival rate overall. And for patients aged 80 or more there was a huge gap in the survival rate (53 per cent compared with the next worst country, Canada, with 68 per cent).[19]

Jacobzone *et al* at the OECD also compared the use of three breast cancer treatments: mastectomy; breast-conserving surgery (BCS); and breast-conserving surgery with post-operative radiation therapy (known as RT after BCS).[20] Since 1985 it has been accepted that RT after BCS has produced a similar survival rate to mastectomy for women diagnosed with early stage breast cancer, whilst avoiding the disfiguring effect of whole breast removal. Nevertheless, rates of BCS as opposed to mastectomy in those aged over 40 vary considerably across countries.[21] In all countries examined by Jacobzone *et al*, treatments varied with increasing age—fewer women 70 years and over received BCS. But the degree of variation in treatments also differs sharply. Patients in Belgium, Canada, France, Italy, Norway and the US received lower levels of BCS in older age groups. In (tax-financed) Sweden and the UK the difference was more stark. Those aged 80+ in Sweden and the UK were half as likely as those aged 70-79 to receive BCS in 1994-5.[22]

Treatment patterns in the UK are singled out for comment by the OECD. Both mastectomy and BCS rates for older women are very low compared to other countries. Jacobzone *et al* show that mastectomy rates tend to rise with age (at least to age 79). However, the UK shows a rate of 11 *per cent* of those 80+ receiving mastectomy, with the average for the eight countries studied being nearly 49 per cent. The UK also has a very low BCS rate for those aged 80+ of only 14 per cent, compared to the average of 28 per cent.[23]

The use of RT after BCS again varies widely from 57 per cent of those receiving BCS in Italy, to 90 *per cent* and 93 *per cent* in Belgium and France respectively. Variation in RT by age is notable in all countries; there is a sharp decline for those over 70. A drop at ages 70-79 occurs in Canada, Italy, Sweden and the UK. However, in Belgium, France and the US patients in that group receive similar treatment to those in younger groups.[24]

A study based on 3.7 million people in Yorkshire found that people over 75 suspected of having cancer were less extensively investigated and, when diagnosed, received less treatment than younger patients. These reductions were not explained by the frailty of patients, nor by the presence of other complicating illnesses.

A study in 1999 found that among the women suspected of having breast cancer, 97 per cent of those under 65 had the diagnosis confirmed by histology (the optimal laboratory test). Among those aged 75 plus it was 63 per cent. Not only were elderly people subject to less thorough *diagnosis*, the optimal *treatment* was often not provided. One per cent of those aged under 65 did not receive the optimal treatment for their clinical condition (in the words of the study, 'no definitive treatment' was provided). However, four per cent of those aged 65-74 failed to receive the optimal treatment; and 11 per cent of those aged 75 plus. Lung cancer sufferers had a similar experience. Of those aged under 65, 80 per cent had their diagnosis confirmed by histology; compared with 70 per cent for the 65-74 year olds; and 44 per cent for those aged 75 plus. And 'no definitive treatment' was provided for 32 per cent of the under 65s, 48 per cent of the 65-74 year olds and 76 per cent of those aged 75 plus.[25]

The simplest explanation for the worrying picture portrayed above, is that some doctors take the view that the elderly have had a 'good innings' and prefer to spend their limited budgets on younger people. This view is reinforced by the tendency to treat individuals as if the average characteristics of their group—the old—applied to every individual. It is accepted by medical ethicists that some treatments can do more harm than good and it is true that the pain and suffering entailed by some medical interventions may outweigh any potential gain. Moreover, at some point death is inevitable and it may be futile to delay it by a few days or weeks. In addition, elderly patients are more likely to have additional complicating illnesses—perhaps both a heart condition and renal failure—and in such circumstances it may be that interventions like renal dialysis and cancer or cardiac surgery will be less effective. But no such conclusion can be drawn in every case. Medical codes of ethics expect decisions to be based on an individual assessment of each patient and the physical condition of people of the same chronological age varies substantially. Medical decisions should, therefore, be based on the individual's unique biological age, not mere chronological age.

Rigid categorisation is not the only problem, however. The underlying cause of age discrimination is that decades of rationing health care have undermined the professional ideal of the doctor as the patient's champion. If there are too few doctors to go round, even the most dedicated will find themselves routinely concocting excuses for not providing clinically necessary treatments.

OECD figures for 2000 show that the UK had 1.8 practising physicians per 1,000 population. Germany had 3.6 per 1,000, France 3.0 and Poland 2.2. The only countries with a lower proportion among the 20 leading nations who supplied information to the OECD were Korea (1.3), and Turkey (1.3).[26] However well motivated individual doctors might be, if they are in short supply, the inevitable result is the dilution of care.

As we get older we tend to need more medical attention, and the chief defence of the NHS is that it will provide care for everyone in their time of need. The unfortunate reality is that is *less* likely to be there just when we need it most.

The American experience

Stephen Pollard

A mericans today are living longer and healthier lives than ever before. By 2030, almost 20 per cent of the US population will be over the age of 65—doubling in number from today to 70 million.

Health experts point to advances in disease treatment and prevention as key factors behind this improvement in the health of older Americans. In recent years, new drugs, medical procedures, screening tools and prevention strategies have improved the treatment of chronic diseases, which affect 80 per cent of all seniors. Prescription drug use has dramatically increased for the elderly, indicating that many are taking advantage of new medicines to improve their health and quality of life; one recent study found that half of the drugs prescribed or administered in doctor's office visits in 1999 did not exist in 1985.[1]

Since 1900, the life expectancy of the average American has increased by 29 years to 79.4 years for females and 73.9 years for males (1999 figures). (The world's population is also ageing. In the next 50 years, the median age of the world's population will increase by 10 years.[2]) Over the past century, and especially in the 1980s and 1990s, the rates of mortality, morbidity and disability among Americans over age 65 have steadily decreased. Between 1979-81 and 1995-97, death rates declined by six per cent in women and 19 per cent in men aged 65 to 74, and eight per cent in women and 16 per cent in men aged 75 to 84.

This paper draws heavily on the US Department of Health and Human Services report, Securing the Benefits of Medical Innovation for Seniors: The Role of Prescription Drugs and Drug Coverage
(http://aspe.hhs.gov/health/reports/medicalinnovation)

Figure 1:1
Percentage of US population aged 65 and older,
1900 - 2050

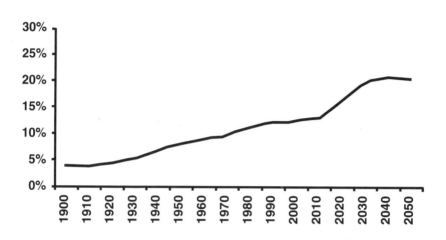

Source: US Census Bureau, Decennial Census Data and Population
Projections

In the past, ageing has been associated with the development of chronic medical conditions, such as cancer, arthritis, diabetes and heart disease, which limit participation in
daily activities and reduce the quality of life. Decreases in
deaths from cardiovascular disease, atherosclerosis, cancer
and hypertension are key contributors to the overall decline
in mortality.

Studies have found that the levels of physical and cognitive disability among older Americans declined during the
1990s, suggesting that seniors are healthier, and more
productive and independent than they were just a decade
ago.[3]

Often, the benefits from development of new drugs and
technologies are additive. For example, a host of medical
advances have combined to yield a 35 per cent reduction in
mortality from coronary heart disease and a 36 per cent
reduction in mortality from stroke since 1980.[4]

In addition to providing cures and preventing more severe and costly effects of diseases, innovations in treatment and medical science, especially pharmaceuticals, have shifted the focus of medicine from highly invasive treatments and surgeries with potentially serious risks to less-invasive practices and therapies focused on prevention and health maintenance. This shift has allowed many older Americans to remain healthy and independent, avoiding long hospital or nursing home stays.

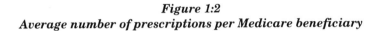

Figure 1:2
Average number of prescriptions per Medicare beneficiary

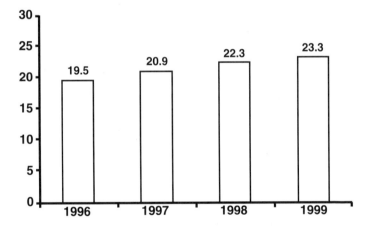

Source: 1999 Medicare Current Beneficiary Survey (MCBS)

Government controls on access to drugs mean that patients who need new therapies often have to wait longer for them or, under cost-containment measures, such as those of the UK's National Institute of Clinical Excellence (NICE), may never have access to them at all. The average time taken for the initial approval and subsequent recognition of a drug by all EU Member States is 643 days. The US average is 335 days.

Many of those over 65 suffer from chronic diseases that have the potential to interfere significantly with their independence and well-being. In the past, as a result of these chronic conditions, many seniors became disabled and were forced to limit their activities. Medical conditions in which recent medical advances have had a dramatic impact on the course of disease and, hence, the quality of individuals' lives include cancer, osteoporosis, asthma, arthritis, high cholesterol, heart attacks, strokes, depression, Alzheimer's disease, type 2 diabetes and migraine. Let us look briefly at the incidence and treatment of these conditions in turn.

Cancer

More than 550,000 Americans die from cancer every year. The US National Cancer Institute estimates that approximately 8.9 million Americans alive today have a history of cancer. Cancer is the second most common cause of death in the United States. Lung, colorectal, prostate and breast cancer are the most common types.

Although there has been an overall decline in US cancer death rates, the cancer burden is expected to rise as the population ages. If the current incidence pattern continues, cancer diagnoses will double from 1.3 million people in 2000 to 2.6 million people in 2050. During this period, the number of cancer patients aged 85 and older is expected to increase four-fold.

Cancer is one of the most expensive diseases to treat. In 2001, total costs for cancer were reported to be in excess of $156 billion, with medical expenditures accounting for approximately $56 billion. Recent advances in biotechnology have yielded some promising new approaches to cancer treatment. But they cost...

Conventional anticancer drugs have tended to be non-selective, attacking both cancerous and healthy cells. Consequently, chemotherapy is often accompanied by a variety of devastating short or long-term side effects. Moreover, individual patient responses to conventional agents are highly variable.

Molecularly targeted therapies based on recent progress in genomics and proteomics, however, hold out the promise of being far more selective, thereby drastically reducing the incidence of side effects in patients undergoing cancer treatment. Gleevec, which is used to treat chronic myeloid leukemia (CML), is one of the first agents using this new approach that targets abnormal proteins fundamental to the cancer. Unlike most current cancer therapies which kill both normal and cancer cells leading to unwanted side-effects, Gleevec and other drugs in this class are designed to zero in on specific cancer-causing molecules, eliminating cancer cells while avoiding serious damage to other, non-cancerous cells. Early studies of this drug have shown that, in patients with CML, white blood-cell counts are restored to normal levels.

And guess what? Although Gleevec is available in the US, you can't have it on the NHS. The National Institute for Clinical Excellence's preliminary review recommended that the drug only be used in patients who had already gone into the 'accelerated phase' of their disease.

Osteoporosis

Ten million Americans have osteoporosis. A further 18 million have low bone mass, placing them at increased risk for the disease. Osteoporosis is responsible for more than 1.5 million fractures per annum—300,000 hip fractures, 700,000 vertebral fractures, 250,000 wrist fractures and more than 300,000 other fractures.

Fifty per cent of women and one out of eight men over 50 will sustain one or more osteoporosis-related fractures of the spine, hip or wrist during their remaining lifetimes. Osteoporosis is thus a major public health threat for 28 million Americans (80 per cent of whom are women). Only one-third of hip fracture patients will return to pre-fracture independence. Estimated direct expenditures (hospitals and nursing homes) for osteoporosis and related fractures are $14 billion per annum.

But effective treatments are available to prevent osteoporosis and reduce the risk of debilitating fractures. Compre-

hensive treatment programmes that focus on proper
nutrition, exercise, medication and prevention of falls, can
slow or stop bone loss, increase bone density and reduce
fracture risk. Bisphosphonates (such as alendronate and
risedronate), first introduced in the mid-1990s, inhibit bone
reabsorption and are one recent category of pharmaceuticals
that effectively treat osteoporosis.

Many countries restrict reimbursement for these drugs to
narrow categories of patients. In Italy, Belgium, and France
only specialists can initiate therapy with Fosamax®, a
bisphosphonate, and then only after the patient has already
suffered one previous, significant osteoporotic fracture and
has a significantly low bone mass density.

Arthritis

Arthritis is the leading cause of disability in the US. One
sixth of the US population (43 million) has arthritis,
limiting the daily activities of seven million people. By 2020,
on current trends, 60 million people will have the disease,
and 11 million will have activity limitations. Forty per cent
of people with arthritis are age 65 or older (see Figure 1:3,
p. 14). Arthritis costs the US nearly $65 billion annually.[5]

Pharmaceuticals are available to control the disabling
symptoms, especially pain, of arthritis. COX-2 inhibitors
interfere with an enzyme that causes pain and swelling.
Moreover, these drugs do not inhibit the COX-1 enzyme,
which may help maintain the normal stomach lining. Thus,
COX-2 inhibitors are reported to have less gastrointestinal
side effects than older drugs, such as aspirin or other non-
steroidal anti-inflammatory agents.

High cholesterol

Approximately 25 per cent of the adult population in the US
has elevated blood cholesterol levels (see Figure 1:4, p. 14).
A high blood cholesterol level is a major risk factor for heart
disease and stroke. Drug therapy can effectively lower blood
cholesterol.

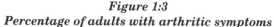

Figure 1:3
Percentage of adults with arthritic symptoms

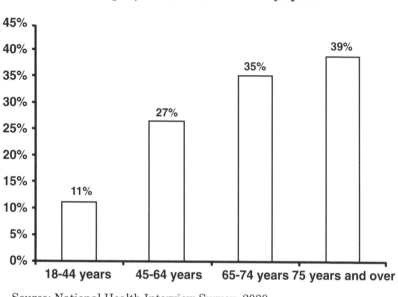

Source: National Health Interview Survey, 2000

Figure 1:4
Percentage of 65-74 year-olds with high serum cholesterol

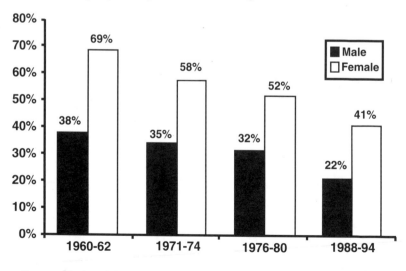

Source: National Health and Nutrition Examination Survey

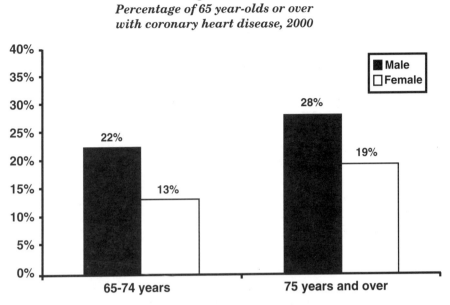

Figure 1:5
Percentage of 65 year-olds or over
with coronary heart disease, 2000

Source: National Health Interview Survey

Since an elevated LDL-cholesterol[6] significantly increases the risk of heart disease, treatment is directed at lowering blood levels. Statins represent a new category of LDL-cholesterol lowering drugs. Their use results in large reductions of total and LDL-cholesterol, which decreases heart attacks and heart disease deaths. Studies using statins have reported 20 to 60 per cent lower LDL-cholesterol levels in patients taking these drugs. Research findings are pointing to other possible benefits of statins: preventing and treating cancer, strokes, Alzheimer's disease, type 2 diabetes, deep vein thrombosis, and organ rejection in transplantation.

Cardiovascular disease—heart disease and stroke

About 950,000 Americans die of cardiovascular disease each year: one death every 33 seconds. Eighty-three per cent of those who die from coronary heart disease are aged 65 or older. Seventy-two per cent of people who suffer a stroke in a given year are 65 or older (see Figure 1:5, p. 15). Heart disease and stroke are respectively the first and third leading causes of death in the United States. They account for more than 40 per cent of deaths.

However, considering deaths alone understates the burden of cardiovascular disease. Sixty-one million Americans (almost a quarter of the population) live with cardiovascular disease. Stroke alone causes the disability of more than four million Americans. Almost six million hospitalisations each year are a result of cardiovascular disease.

Strokes and heart attacks have a higher incidence rate in those aged 65 and over. High blood pressure and diabetes are chronic conditions that predispose individuals to develop cardiovascular disease. Both diseases have a relatively high prevalence in that age group.

Recently developed treatments for heart attacks and strokes have reduced morbidity and improved mortality. Tissue Plasminogen Activator (t-PA) is a thrombolytic agent, known as a 'clot-busting' drug. It can dissolve blood clots, which cause most heart attacks and strokes. The prompt use (within the first three hours) of t-PA following an ischaemic stroke has been shown to halt damage and significantly improve recovery. In addition, prompt treatment of stroke victims with t-PA could result in substantial net cost savings to the health care system. t-PA-treated stroke patients, because of their decreased disability, leave hospital sooner and require less rehabilitation and nursing after discharge than patients who do not receive t-PA.

Advances in medical science have yielded new approaches to the treatment of cardiovascular disease. The Pharmaceutical Research Manufacturers of America (PhRMA) reports that 122 new medicines were in development for cardiovascular diseases in 2002. Some of these new agents are directed at chronic medical conditions that are risk factors for the development of heart disease, such as high blood pressure or high cholesterol. Others are new treatments for complications of heart disease.

There are essentially two complementary strategies under development, aimed at reducing morbidity from a stroke. One is to restore blood flow to the brain as quickly as possible; the second is to limit the damage incurred by a stroke.

Research is underway on a clot-dissolving drug made from the venom of a pit viper snake. While this drug has not yet been approved, early findings suggest that it helps stroke patients regain their physical and mental abilities, with many patients experiencing full recovery.

Depression

Six per cent of Americans aged 65 and older in a given year (approximately 2 million of the 34 million such adults), have a diagnosable depressive illness. As a result of depression, older Americans are disproportionately likely to commit suicide. Although they comprise only 13 per cent of the US population, individuals aged 65 and older accounted for 19 per cent of all suicide deaths in 1997. Major depression is a leading cause of disability.

In contrast to the normal emotional experiences of sadness, grief, loss or passing mood states, depressive disorders can be extreme and persistent and can significantly interfere with an individual's ability to function. Depression often co-occurs with other illnesses such as cardiovascular disease, stroke, diabetes and cancer, which have a significant incidence in seniors. When depression co-occurs with such medical conditions, it can interfere with the patient's ability to follow the necessary treatment regimen or to participate in a rehabilitation programme. Depression may also increase impairment from the medical disorder and impede its improvement.

Anti-depressants are widely used, effective treatments for depression. Existing anti-depressant drugs are known to influence the functioning of certain neurotransmitters in the brain, primarily serotonin and norepinephrine. Older medications—tricyclic anti-depressants and monoamine oxidase inhibitors—affect the activity of both of these neurotransmitters simultaneously. The disadvantage of these older medications is that they can be difficult to tolerate owing to side effects or dietary and/or medication restrictions. Newer medications, such as the selective serotonin reuptake inhibitors (SSRIs), have significantly fewer side effects than older drugs, making it easier for patients, including older adults, to adhere to treatment. Other recently introduced anti-depressants may be better tolerated by patients suffering from depression.

Alzheimer's disease

An estimated four million Americans have Alzheimer's disease. Approximately ten per cent of people older than 65 years, and 47 per cent of those older than 85 years, have the disease (see Figure 1:6, below). The death rate for people with Alzheimer's disease is twice as high as the rate among those of the same age without the disease. The prevalence of Alzheimer's doubles every five years after 65.

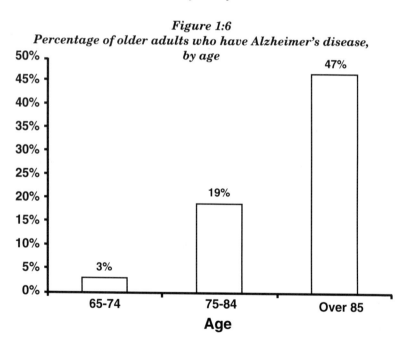

Figure 1:6
Percentage of older adults who have Alzheimer's disease, by age

Source: Evans, D. *et al*, *Journal of the American Medical Association*, vol. 262, no. 18, 1989.

Because the risk of Alzheimer's disease increases with age, the prevalence of the disease is anticipated to increase as the US population ages. This will incur a substantial economic and social burden. The estimated annual economic toll of healthcare expenses owing to Alzheimer's patients and caregivers in the US is currently $80 to $100 billion. This estimate includes both direct and indirect costs for medical and long-term care, home care and loss of productivity for caregivers.

According to PhRMA, over 20 clinical trials of new drugs to treat Alzheimer's disease were underway in 2001. Antioxidants and anti-inflammatory agents are being tested for effectiveness in treating Alzheimer's disease. A compound that activates neural growth factors in the brain is being tested. A drug that increases signaling between nerve cells is also under study.

Diabetes

Seventeen million Americans have diabetes. Over 200,000 people die each year from complications related to the disease. Diabetes afflicts approximately 20 per cent of all Americans age 65 and older. The elderly with diabetes often experience a reduced quality of life. Diabetes incurs a tremendous personal, social and financial burden. In 1997, for persons aged 65 and older, total direct medical expenditures attributable to diabetes in the US exceeded $32 billion. The high price of diabetes includes frequent physician and emergency room visits and admissions to hospitals and nursing homes.

Optimal treatment of diabetes can improve the quality of life and reduce health care costs. Clinical trials have shown that intensive control of blood glucose, blood pressure and lipids can dramatically reduce the risk of complications. Many patients initially control their diabetes with diet and exercise. Oral hypoglycemics are one popular form of drug treatment for type 2 diabetes. Ultimately, most patients will require insulin. Improved formulations of insulin and methods of insulin delivery are currently in development. Treatment with hypoglycemic agents may prevent individuals from developing diabetes.

In the Diabetes Prevention Program, a clinical trial involving over 3,000 people at high risk for type 2 diabetes, diet and exercise that achieved a five to seven per cent weight loss reduced diabetes incidence by 58 per cent. Treatment with metformin reduced the risk of developing diabetes in individuals at high risk for type 2 diabetes by 31 per cent over 2.8 years. Starch blockers, which delay the digestion and absorption of sugars from food, were also demonstrated to cut the odds that high-risk adults would develop diabetes by 25 per cent over three years.

In 2002, 23 drugs were in clinical trials for the treatment and prevention of diabetes.

Conclusion

Current US senior citizens are the beneficiaries of medical innovations that have dramatically improved their quality of life in their golden years. With the recent discoveries in medical science, future breakthroughs in treating and curing chronic diseases are probable.

To ensure continued progress in the fight to treat and prevent chronic disease, society must provide a nurturing environment in which research and development can flourish.

Efforts to encourage medical innovations should include investing in biomedical research, protecting intellectual property rights, providing for an efficient regulatory process and fairly compensating industry for its products.

We should recognise that the pre-eminence of the US in pharmaceuticals, the treatment given to its seniors and the benefits of a health system are not mere co-incidences but are inter-related. We should similarly ponder the relationship between the state of British treatment of its pensioners and the NHS.

Cancer care: a bottomless pit?

Karol Sikora

Introduction

Cancer is an emotive business in current society. Increasingly common as our populations get older, it now affects one in three and will affect one in two in the next decade. It is not one but many diseases arising in different parts of the body because of mutations and functional abnormalities in the intricate molecular machinery that controls normal growth, cell division and death in our cells. Lung, prostate, breast and colorectal cancers make up over 60 per cent of the disease burden but there are 202 separate cancer types, all with many subdivisions in terms of optimal treatment and outcome.

Treatment usually involves surgery or radiotherapy to deal with the primary site of the disease and chemotherapy —treatment with drugs—to control disease that has spread. Patients are now fully informed of their diagnosis and are given huge amounts of information about their own illness. In addition the world-wide-web hosts over 15 million cancer sites. With best available treatment, around 45 per cent of patients will be completely cured and another 30 per cent have meaningful prolongation of survival. All will gain at least palliative benefit in terms of symptom improvement and increased physical comfort.

But treatment is expensive. As it becomes more effective, with more precise computerised radiotherapy delivery and new molecularly targeted drugs, the financial envelopes of most healthcare delivery systems, including the NHS in Britain, will become increasingly stretched. Here, I will examine the likely future of cancer care from both a technological and societal viewpoint. Figure 2:1 (p. 22) examines the components of the cancer future.

21

22

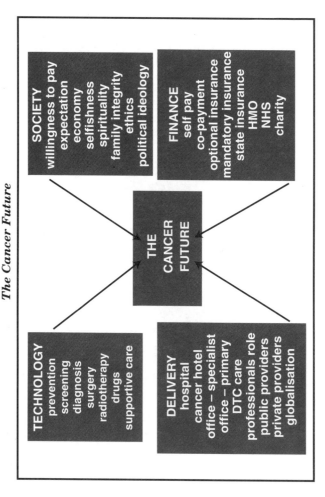

Figure 2:1
The Cancer Future

Source: Modified from Sikora, K., 'The impact of future technology on cancer care', *Clinical Medicine*, 2: 560-68, 2002.

Figure 2:2
Alternative Cancer Futures

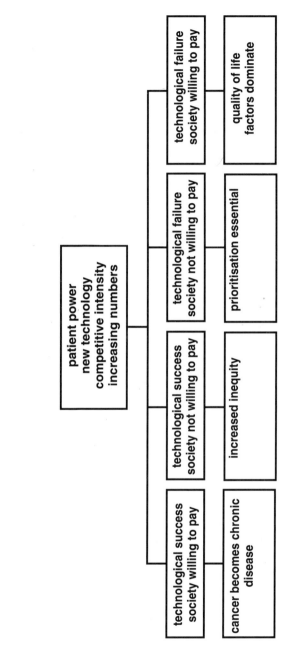

Source: Modified from Sikora, K., 'The impact of future technology on cancer care', *Clinical Medicine*, 2: 560-68, 2002.

Alternative futures

The cancer future is made up of four components. Technology will inexorably improve although the pace is difficult to predict. The human genome project, the power of modern molecular biology and the number-crunching ability of bioinformatics have given us a new understanding of cancer and how to develop very selective drugs to inhibit its growth.

Technology clearly costs and society needs to examine how much it is willing to pay for any benefit. Implicit but unpopular is the concept of rationing in healthcare. Politicians of all leanings are well aware that the 'R' word is a vote loser. Complex mechanisms are in place to ensure rationing without overt discussion. In the UK the National Institute of Clinical Excellence (NICE) assesses therapies and provides guidelines for their use. There is some consistency emerging with the upper cost limit for extending life by one year being placed at £35,000. Such cost-benefit analyses are by no means an exact science. There is also good evidence of continued postcode prescribing with inconsistency in enacting guidelines across small geographical areas. Vocal, well-educated patients are more likely to access expensive therapies that those from less privileged backgrounds.

The third component of the future is the delivery mechanism. Hospitals will transform into far friendlier hotel-like environments over the next decade. Cancer will become like diabetes today—a chronic, controllable illness managed by relatively non-toxic medication requiring frequent monitoring and adjustment.

Perhaps the biggest challenge will be the financial model underpinning cancer care. We simply can't believe the politicians' lies. But we have to pay the price somehow—through taxation, insurance or directly.

The consistent strands in the future of cancer care are increasing patient power and lobbying; new technology with step changes that are difficult to predict; increased competitive intensity in the commercial development of new cancer treatments; and increasing numbers of patients as diagnostic techniques improve and the population ages. There are essentially four potential futures depending on the relative success of technology in prolonging survival and the willingness of society to pay for its implementation (Figure 2:2, p. 23).

In the most favourable, technological success is delivered rapidly and society is willing to pay for it, making cancer a chronic, controllable disease by 2020. In the second, society is not willing to pay—leading to increasing inequity with the rich getting more effective care than the poor. This scenario would be similar to the current situation with HIV-related disease in Africa. The other two alternatives assume little technological advance. Here quality of life improvements arising from effective palliation dominate in therapy choice provided society is willing to pay for them. In poor environments a fourth future of rigid prioritisation to maximise therapeutic gain will become essential although inequity will abound. It is likely that the real future will be a mixture of boxes one and two—with technological success and partial funding for a potentially bottomless pit.

Technological future

Surgery

Cancer surgery has been a dramatic success. Effective cancer surgery began in the late nineteenth century when it was realised that tumours could be removed along with their regional lymph nodes. This enhanced the chances of complete cure as it had the greatest possibility of avoiding any spread of the cancer. Surgery still remains the single most effective modality for cancer treatment. Increasingly it has become far more conservative, able to retain organs and structures. Breast cancer is an excellent example. The radical mastectomy performed until 30 years ago left women with severe deformity on the chest wall. This was replaced firstly by the less mutilating simple mastectomy and now by excision biopsy followed by radiotherapy. The breast remains fully intact.

New technology already permits minimally invasive (keyhole) surgery for many cancer types. The science of robotics will allow completely automated surgical approaches with enhanced effects and minimal damage to surrounding structures. Ultimately, it is likely surgery will disappear as an important treatment and become confined simply to biopsy performed under local anaesthetic with image guidance to check that the correct site is identified. Although this will reduce the duration and costs of hospital admission, it is likely that cost of developing and maintaining the necessary expertise will remain extremely high, indeed similar to current conventional surgical costs.

Radiotherapy

Radiotherapy was first used for cancer treatment over a hundred years ago. Originally crude radium was used as the radiation source, but we now have a variety of sophisticated techniques available. Modern linear accelerators—the workhorse for radiotherapy—allow precise dose delivery precisely to the shape of the tumour. Conformal therapy aims to deliver high doses to the tumour volume in three dimensions, killing the cancer cells and avoiding sensitive normal surrounding tissue. Novel computer-based imaging techniques have revolutionised our ability to understand the precise anatomy of cancer in a patient and therefore to deliver far more effective radiotherapy. The future of radiotherapy is further computerisation with multimedia imaging and optimised conformal planning. We have also learned to understand the biological differences among different tumours in patients and can begin to plan individualised treatment courses to optimise selective destruction. Future radiotherapy is likely to involve increasingly expensive technology to ensure precise delivery—potentially doubling its current costs.

Chemotherapy

Chemotherapy began after the sinking of an American battleship in Bari Harbour, Italy in 1943. It was noticed that leucopenia developed in many of the injured. Although shrouded in secrecy at the time, alkylating agents for use as chemical warfare agents were being carried. This led naval physicians to treat patients with lymphoma and leukaemia with nitrogen mustard. A new era of cancer care had begun.

Table 2:1
Cancer chemosensitivity groups

Chemotherapy for advanced cancer
November 2002

high CR	high CR	low CR
high cure	low cure	low cure
5%	40%	55%
HD	AML	NSCLC
ALL	breast	colon
testis	ovary	stomach
chorio	SCLC	prostate
childhood	sarcoma	pancreas
BL	myeloma	glioma

Source: Modified from Sikora, K., 'The impact of future technology on cancer care', *Clinical Medicine*, 2: 560-68, 2002.

There are three groups of cancers in terms of chemosensitivity (Table 2:1). In the first, we can achieve a high complete response rate and a high cure rate. These include Hodgkin's disease, childhood leukaemia and other cancers, choriocarcinoma and testicular cancer. Unfortunately, this group of successfully treated cancers represents less than five per cent of the global cancer burden. At the other end we have a group with a low complete response and low cure rate such as lung, colon and stomach cancer. So far chemotherapy has made little inroads, although some useful palliation and prolongation of survival sometimes for months can be achieved. In the middle there are cancers with a high complete response but a low cure rate. These cause problems in resource allocation. The use of taxanes in breast and ovarian cancer is a classic example. Here, high-cost drugs can achieve extension of life by several months for many patients. When deciding on priorities we have to assess how much we are willing to pay for a month of reasonable quality life. The NHS currently limits this to about £1,000 for cancer, although nowhere is this figure openly discussed. Rationing is deplored by patients, support groups and politicians but also used relentlessly by the media to demonstrate the inadequacies of the system.

Drug discovery and development

Cancer drug development is entering a remarkable new phase. Recent advances in molecular biology have led to a host of new, validated targets. In silico drug design allows the construction of thousands of virtual compounds, the most promising of which can be rapidly synthesised. This complements robotic high throughput screening of well organised chemical and natural compound libraries. This has led to a platform approach to drug discovery—the creation of specific inhibitors for each member of a gene family such as the protein kinases. This approach has been remarkably successful and a range of small molecules are now available that affect processes as diverse as cell cycle control, mitotic spindle separation, apoptosis, signal transduction, angiogenesis and tumour invasion. Over the last five years there has been a shift away from the search for new cytotoxic drugs to drugs acting through defined molecular mechanisms known to be aberrant in cancer. There are currently nearly 500 molecules undergoing clinical study and this may well reach 1,000 by 2004. Clearly, new methods to identify and prioritise the most promising candidates are necessary, as there are only limited resources to take these compounds into expensive and time consuming phase III studies. Figure 2:3 (p. 30) shows the potential timeline for the introduction of new technology to the marketplace. The critical years are predicted to be 2005-10.

Molecular profiling is the holistic profiling of a tumour using several technologies to determine its likely natural history and optimal therapy. The beginnings of such correlations have been used in assays for the expression of specific gene products in increased, reduced or mutated form. Examples include erbB1, erbB2, ras and p53. The emerging technologies of genomics, proteomics and metabonomics can produce enormous datasets to correlate with tumour behaviour patterns and response to different therapies. Although current data are fascinating, it will take several years before 'personalised medicine' becomes a reality for the majority of cancer patients. By 2030 it is likely that near patient testing using 'black box' systems will guide therapy choice by computer print-out.

All of these innovations have a price tag. Increasingly, the commercialisation of drugs involves ways to maximise their life cycle and defend them from generic competition. Innovation is the key to success, as smart marketers can always create a demand for the new, even if the gain is tiny. Direct to consumer advertising, support for patient advocacy groups, defending high cost branded drugs against generics and changing physicians' mindsets by sophisticated promotional activities create a huge sink for healthcare funding.

Supportive care

The hospice movement has injected a much needed sense of reality into the much hyped world of cancer drug development. Immortality is simply unachievable. We need to encourage society to provide novel care structures within the community, as close to patients' homes as possible. Mood control drugs may remove the depression sometimes associated with terminal illness. In seeking to achieve compressed morbidity it is likely that euthanasia will become formalised. Seamlessness between cancer treatment and supportive care will become emphasised as part of a far more integrated, holistic and patient-focused package delivered in attractive hotel-like environments that deliberately downplay technology.

But tender loving care costs money. As people live longer with their cancer, they will require more care in late life. The role of women in society has changed dramatically over the last 50 years which taken together with the decline in family integrity and increased mobility has led to a huge care problem, not just for cancer patients. Care of the chronically ill was traditionally undertaken by family groups—led by women. This is no longer possible in many families.

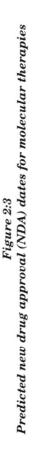

Figure 2:3
Predicted new drug approval (NDA) dates for molecular therapies

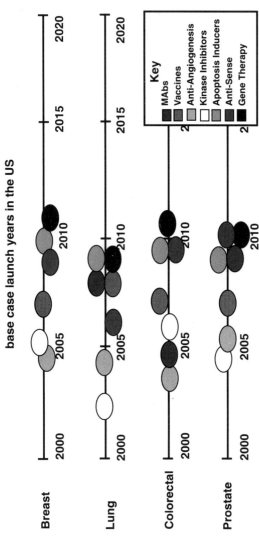

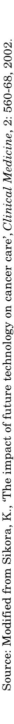

Figure 2:4
The cancer demand pyramid in 2010

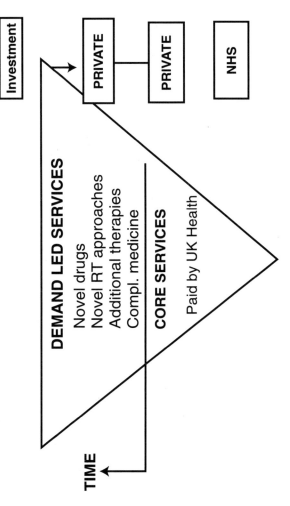

Source: Modified from Sikora, K., 'The impact of future technology on cancer care', *Clinical Medicine*, 2: 560-68, 2002.

32

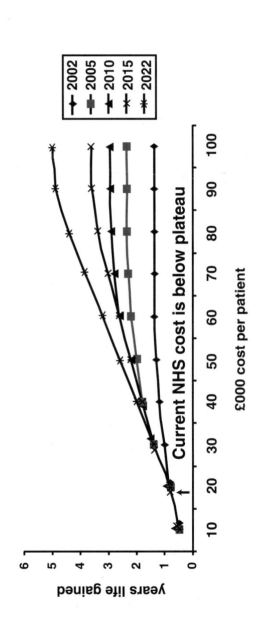

Figure 2:5
The cost of innovation on an individual patient basis

Source: Modified from Sikora, K., 'The impact of future technology on cancer care', *Clinical Medicine*, 2: 560-68, 2002.

Cancer services in Britain

How will cancer services in Britain evolve? The National Cancer Plan is delivering increasing funding and significant improvements in infrastructure although there are many examples where the promised extra funding has simply been lost in the morass of NHS administration. The 2003 figure for extra funds for cancer is £504 million. But this does not take into account salary increases, EU work directives, new appraisal systems and new working practices that will considerably reduce the actual money available.

But there is good evidence that even this seemingly massive injection of funds will never keep up with demand. Complex assessments of cost-effectiveness fail to reassure patients seeking cure at any price. Organisations such as NICE will never convince determined and organised patient groups that in the end their deliberations are not a form of rationing. The pressures to expand demand are driven by potential financial gain by the pharmaceutical and healthcare industry and fanned by the media's insatiable appetite for controversy. What politician can afford to be seen to condone the refusal of a new drug for a young woman with breast cancer, pictured with her two beautiful children on the front of a national newspaper?

Figure 2:4 (p. 31) illustrates the dilemma of the cancer demand pyramid. However generous the core services, there will be an increase in demand led services that will remain outside the core package. These demands may be for new, high-cost drugs with marginal benefit, more precise radiotherapy technology, complementary medicines, or simply better hotel facilities in hospital. Some form of co-payment model is inevitable in their provision. The private sector can provide many demand led services unavailable in the NHS. As public and private services move closer to a unified provider model, a more transparent allocation of resources is now needed to avoid the pressures imposed by postcode prescribing and other geographic inconsistencies.

Figure 2:5 (p. 32) examines the cost of innovation on an individual patient basis. The lower curve is for 2002. As more money is spent on an individual we get up to a plateau of efficacy limited by the success of current technology. As we move through the next 20 years it is likely that the treatment of cancer will significantly improve. By 2022 the plateau will be much higher—it may cost up to £100,000 in today's currency to treat a cancer patient optimally.

There is good evidence that the NHS operates below the optimal funding level. For this reason our cancer survival rates are poorer than those in many European countries. Ministers may try to disguise the fact that our overall cancer mortality is lower, largely thanks to better tobacco control 30 years ago, but once cancer actually occurs, the chances of it being successfully treated are still significantly lower than in mainland Europe.

Conclusion

We urgently need to ensure open and mature debate about the best way to deal with the financial consequences of cancer if we are to avoid sinking huge healthcare resources into a bottomless pit. Table 2:2 examines the features of cancer care in 2022.

Table 2:2
Providing Cancer Care in 2022

- Cancer becomes a chronic controllable disease
- 'Cancer hotels' in most towns
- New roles for cancer professionals
- Negotiators to help with options
- Black box near patient testing systems to guide therapy
- Novel financial, insurance delivery systems
- Global provider franchises

Source: Modified from Sikora, K., 'The impact of future technology on cancer care', *Clinical Medicine*, 2: 560-68, 2002.

Getting there will involve huge shifts in the NHS. Health care began as a charity often with a religious background. The names of the great London teaching hospitals are mainly those of saints; the inception of the NHS in postwar Britain brought an era of militaristic hierarchy. We are now in a systems-focused, Stalinist period with collaboratives, networks, commissioners and modernisation plans with strict central control and a massive propaganda machine that tries to suppress deviant behaviour such as writing this article. Health care's journey will inevitably take it to where it belongs—a customer focused, easy to use, consumer responsive system. The delivery of cancer care will be no exception.

Population ageing:
challenge and response

John Grimley Evans

The challenge

Ageing is a universal, biological phenomenon character-ised by loss of adaptability by individual organisms as time passes. It is this loss of adaptability that underlies the characteristics of illnesses in old age that need to be planned for in the design of our healthcare systems (Table 3:1). They dictate the need for appropriate systems of health care, not just a congeries of independent specialties. This has been known for forty years but many centres in the UK are still waiting.

Table 3:1
Characteristics of disease in later life

- Multiple pathology
- Cryptic or non-specific presentation
- Rapid deterioration if untreated
- High incidence of secondary complications
- Vulnerability to adverse environment
- Need for active rehabilitation

Even if we did not age, we would still all die eventually from disease, famine, accident, predation or warfare, but our risk of dying would remain constant with age or even decline owing to natural selection for the fittest. In the human species, death rates are high in early childhood and fall to a nadir around the age of ten when senescence first emerges in a rise with age in total mortality rates (Figure 3:1, p. 37). After perturbations in early adult life due to violent deaths, mortality rates rise as a more or less exponential function of age throughout the rest of the lifespan. The slope of the exponential function linking mortality and age remains remarkably constant, despite large differences in the level of mortality rates.[1] The point of lowest mortality has also remained constant around 10 to 11 in England for over a hundred years (Figure 3:2, p. 38).[2]

Interacting with the intrinsic genetic processes that set the basic pattern of ageing are extrinsic factors in environment and lifestyle. Comparison of the expectation of life at ages through the lifespan of women in the nineteenth and late twentieth centuries shows that the proportional increase in expectation has been remarkable similar throughout adult ages. The percentage increase in expectancy at age 100 has been the same as at age 30 or 40 (Figure 3:3, p. 38, note semilogarithmic plot).

Figure 3:1
Mortality and age

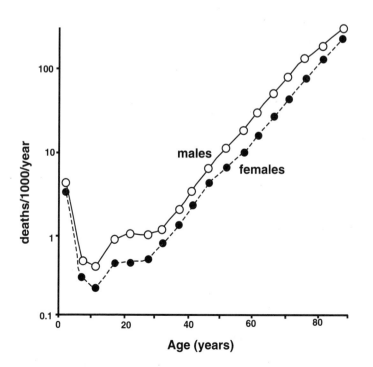

Figure 3:2
Age of lowest mortality

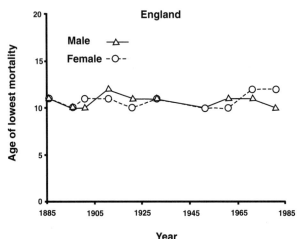

Source: Grimley Evans, 1997.[2]

Figure 3:3
***Life expectancy, England, females,
1871-80 and 1980-82 logarithmic scale***

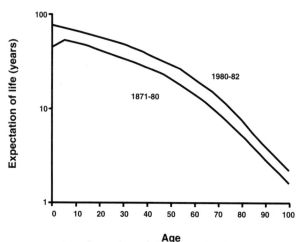

Source: Grimley Evans, 1997.[2]

Figure 3:4
Fertility and child mortality rates over time

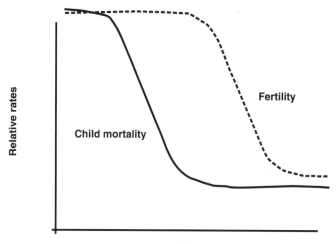

Figure 3:5
Population structures of 1901 and 1971

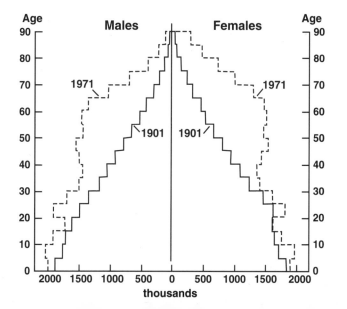

Figure 3:6
Projected number of older people sufficiently
disabled to need daily personal help

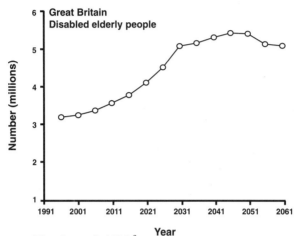

Source: Martin *et al*, 1988.[3]

Figure 3:7
Numbers of people of working age
in the population over time

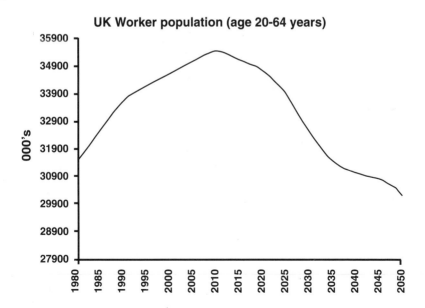

Increased life expectancy is only one source of older people. In recent times another has been the so-called demographic transition. As nations undergo economic development there comes a point when for reasons that are not always clear, and probably vary from place to place, child mortality rates start to fall. There is then a gap, typically of at least a generation, before fertility rates and family sizes fall (Figure 3:4, p. 39). There is therefore a bolus of unprecedented survivors of childhood released into the population to swell the numbers of older people seven or eight decades later. The British demographic transition took place in the early years of the twentieth century, and the effects can be seen in a comparison of the population structures of 1901 and 1971 (Figure 3:5, p. 39). The products of the demographic transition are now passing through the last years of their lives, but a second wave of population ageing will arise from the baby boomers of the high birth rates in the 1950s. Figure 3:6 (p. 40) shows the numbers of older people sufficiently disabled to need personal help in activities of daily living that we can expect if disability rates in old age remain at today's levels. We will need to organise care for another two million people.

The full significance of this emerges if we view the numbers of people of working age in the population over the relevant period (Figure 3:7, p. 40). The need for personal care will reach a peak as the number of people available to provide the care is approaching its lowest.

The response
What are we trying to achieve?

There are four elements in formulating a response.
Population ageing: four imperatives:

- Decide what we are trying to achieve
- Identify funding needs and sources
- Improve efficiency of services
- Reduce need for services

Obviously, the first is to decide what we are trying to achieve. Here it is logical to ask older people what they want from life. Independence and dignity figure high in their priorities as exemplified in the comments of one of my elderly patients: 'I do not mind being old and everyone has got to die; but I do not want to be a burden'. Young people, asked about their own future old age, give very similar answers. The priority target is to prevent disability, and the dependency and indignity it may bring.

Funding

Two main methods of funding in place around the world are the 'pay-as-you-go' system in which people currently working are paying for those currently needing care, and an insurance model in which individuals accumulate resources on which they have a right to draw in times of need. Pay-as-you-go is more efficient as there are fewer middlemen taking their cuts, and it automatically underwrites inflation. But it raises the problem of intergenerational equity when, as we have seen to be the case in Britain, successive generations are of very different sizes. Insurance models can seem in this situation to be more equitable although as Eatwell has shown, in terms of their impact on the economy, they are necessarily equivalent.[4] Both require the sequestration of resources for one generation from another.

For whatever reasons, pensions are being increasingly established on an insurance model. There is no doubt that increasing longevity will require pensions to be met by longer working lives and higher or subsidised contributions. Quick fixes the by mass immigration of workers are a recipe for social misery and only postpone the problem, for young immigrants become old pensioners.

Consequences for health costs from population ageing have been greatly exaggerated by a misunderstanding of the data. In cross-sectional data (Figure 3:8, p. 43), costs per head per year rise steeply on average in later life. Longitudinal data, as compiled by Zweifel *et al* (Figure 3:9, p. 44),[5] show that most of our lifetime healthcare costs are crammed into the last months of life. They are in fact the costs of dying and have to be incurred at whatever age we die. Indeed, in American data, the older people are when they set about dying, the less the process costs. The rise in average cost with age in cross-sectional data is simply due to the fact that the older the age group studied, the higher the proportion of individuals going through the business of dying. Zweifel calculates that the impact of ageing on USA healthcare costs is negligible; it is unjust and unconstructive to make older people the scapegoats for escalation in costs.

Figure 3:8
Healthcare costs per capita per year

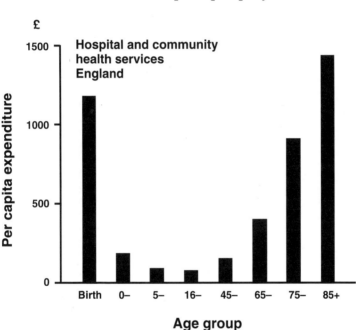

Efficiency of health services

Improving the efficiency of health services is the third of our imperatives and one that is a widespread preoccupation of researchers and policy makers. Evidence-based medicine is an overvalued approach to the issue, but good sense may yet prevail.[6]

Figure 3:9

Healthcare expenditure over last year of life, people aged 65+

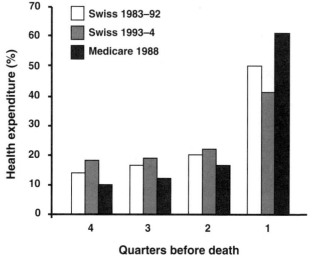

Source: Zweifel *et al*, 1999.[5]

Figure 3:10

Observed older people with disability in the USA, and expected number of older disabled, had rates stayed at the 1982 levels

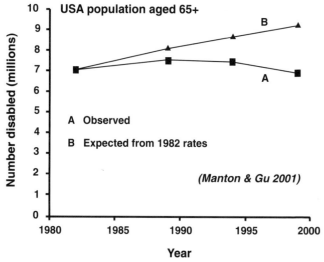

Source: Manton and Gu, 2001.[7]

Reducing the need for services

We have paid less attention to reducing the need for services, and yet it is perhaps the most effective response to population ageing. Recent American experience suggests that we do not have to accept present patterns of disability in old age as inevitable. Since the 1980s, the US has conducted a series of health interviews and examinations of nationally representative samples of the population. Over that period the longevity of the older members of the American population has increased, but the prevalence of disability in the population aged over 65 has been falling. There are now two million fewer older people with disability in the USA than would have been expected if rates had stayed at the levels they were in 1982 (Figure 3:10, p. 44). There are no European data of a quality comparable with those of the USA, so we do not know if the same is happening on this side of the Atlantic, although there is a suggestion that it may be happening in the Netherlands. It is important that we do not let politicians make the convenient (for them) assumption that what has been happening in the US will necessarily happen elsewhere. The point is that because the changes in the USA must be largely extrinsic in origin the same could be made to happen elsewhere.

Essentially we want to live longer but to die faster, and Table 3:2 (below) lists the ways the USA have probably achieved this and how we could go about it.

Table 3:2
Living longer, dying faster

- Postponement as prevention
  - Lifestyle
  - Knowledge, opportunities, incentives
  - Public health and medical care
- Disability-reducing interventions
- Less disabling environments
  - Less poverty
  - Architecture and planning

Biologically, a key approach is through postponement as prevention. Because of age-associated loss of adaptability the older we are when struck by a potentially disabling disease such as stroke or coronary disease, the more likely we are to die from it rather than linger in a disabled state. Postponing disease is partly a matter of lifestyle—boring old things like exercising, not smoking, eating a sensible diet. But healthy lifestyles are a societal as well as an individual issue. We have concentrated too much on health education as a means of persuading people to live healthier lives; health education increases knowledge but rarely changes behaviour. We should think more about opportunities and incentives, such as making cities safer and more pleasant for pedestrians and cyclists rather than car drivers, and persuading supermarkets to take their profits from junk foods while subsidising fruit and vegetables.

A second element in postponement as prevention lies with the medical aspects of preventive medicine. Both primary and secondary prevention have lower priority in our health systems than they merit, and older people are often excluded. One reason is the dominance of monetary considerations in the thinking of politicians. We now have good reason to believe that benefit from drugs such as statins and ACE-inhibitors extend to a much wider range of preventive contexts than emerged from their earlier use in high-risk conditions. Perhaps we cannot afford to hand them out unrestrictedly through health services, but have we really thought through the implications of a democratic commitment to the freedom of choice of an informed public? People are free to spend money on cigarettes if they choose. Could they be given greater personal choice over spending their money on preventive medicine through medically sanctioned over-the-counter purchase?

One reason for the under use of preventive treatments for older people is the assumption that such interventions will be less effective in later life. In fact, older people will commonly benefit more than do younger. This is to be expected on biological grounds. Effective treatments typically reduce the risk of death or undesirable outcome in a probabilistic fashion manifested in a percentage reduction of the background (untreated) risk. Because of age-associated loss of adaptability, the background risk rises with age and x per cent of a large number is greater than x per cent of a smaller. So the number of lives saved or undesirable outcomes prevented per thousand patients treated will rise with age. As an exemplar, Table 3:3 (below) presents data from a trial of beta-blockers after myocardial infarction, and Table 3:4 (below) lists some of the treatments for which enhanced effect at older ages has been shown. Note that these interventions are used not just to prevent death but also to prevent disabling conditions such as stroke and heart attacks.

Table 3:3
Fatality rates in patients treated with beta-blockers after myocardial infarction

Timolol after myocardial infarction

Fatality rates

Age	Control (%)	Reduction (%)	Lives saved per 1,000
<65	9.7	48.4	47
65-	15.3	47.7	73

Source: The Norwegian Multicentre Study Group, 1981.[8]

Table 3:4
Treatments for which enhanced effect at older ages has been shown

Treatments with greater absolute effect at older ages than in younger patients

- Thrombolysis (selection necessary?)
- Statins
- Beta-blockers
- Aspirin
- ACE inhibitors
- Hypotensives

The next item on the agenda is the rational deployment of disability-reducing interventions. Rehabilitation after acute illness in old age is one crucial element provided best by specialist departments of geriatrics. But there are many others. For older people there is a striking disparity between the levels of provision of disability-reducing interventions such as coronary artery surgery and angioplasty and joint replacements in the USA and Britain (Table 3:5, below). And this comparison makes no account of the higher prevalence of disability consequent on long waiting times in the UK.

Table 3:5
Disability-reducing interventions,
rates* per 100,000, people aged 75 and over,
USA 1995, England 1999

	USA	England	Ratio
Hip replacement	860	434	2
Knee replacement	452	304	1.5
CABG	320	57	5.3
Coronary angioplasty	307	40	7.7
Carotid endarterectomy	287	34	8.4

* Standardised for sex and age group

Finally, we need to consider the implications of the fact that disability arises when there is an ecological gap between what our environment demands of us and what we are capable of doing.[9] An unsuitable environment can be as damaging as a person's physical or mental impairment. Quality of housing and household equipment are matters related to personal wealth. But at a societal level, architects and planners are not sufficiently aware of the design implications of the needs of increasing numbers of older people in our populations. Too many roads are impossible for local resident to cross, even where it is essential for them to do so in order to do basic shopping. There are a few research teams working on non-disabling environments but the design requirements they specify are not written routinely into briefs for architects and planners as they should be.

The central challenge in the agenda presented is that it calls for a system rather than piecemeal interventions, and for long-term strategies rather than the quick fixes and ministerial initiatives beloved of modern politicians and their propagandists. The lack of serious governmental response to the Carnegie Inquiry Report on the Third Age[10] suggests that we lack the political machinery necessary for rising to the challenge. The initiative may lie with older people themselves. They comprise a sufficient percentage of the electorate to be able to change the natural course of political events if they could learn to vote tactically. Much of what has happened in the USA was achieved through older people's voting power and the determination of organisations such as the grey panthers. Perhaps this is something else we might usefully learn from American experience.

Direct and indirect constraints on commissioning of specialist medical care

Roger Williams

My aim in this presentation is to describe the constraints currently placed on the commissioning of specialised medical care, which inevitably leads to a rationing of it. I am going to take examples from my own field of liver disease and in doing so will also indicate whether elderly patients are being particularly affected and how the limits are being imposed.

Sadly, with respect to liver disease in the UK, both morbidity and mortality figures are increasing. This was one of the important messages of the Chief Medical Officer (CMO) in his annual report for 2001. Mortality had increased seven times for males and eight times for females over the past 30 years. The CMO was particularly concerned over the increased number of deaths in the working- age groups but looking at the figures from the perspective of today's symposium, it is to be noted that some one third of the mortality was in subjects aged 65 years or more. As indicated in Table 4:1 (p. 51), the statistics show a substantial burden on hospital services in terms of the number of admissions and bed-days usage. As pointed out in the Royal College of Physicians Report, there are also a substantial number of patients admitted to hospital with unrelated conditions who are heavy drinkers in whom there may be an

I am grateful to Dr Barbara Gill of London RSCG for much helpful information on the work of the RSCG and the National Specialised Services Definitions Set.

opportunity at that time to address the situation and prevent additional medical illnesses.[1]

Table 4:1
The rising tide of liver disease in the UK

- *CMO's Report 2001* - over 4,000 deaths from cirrhosis in 1999. Two thirds before 65th birthday. Mortality (x7 for males, 8 for females) over past 30 years. Cirrhosis kills more men than Parkinson's disease and more women than cancer of the cervix.

- *Hospital Episodes 2000 / 01*
  Over 15,000 admissions for alcoholic liver disease (129,000 bed days), almost 4,000 for fibrosis/ cirrhosis (25,000 bed days), 3,000 for chronic viral hepatitis, and over 5,000 for malignant neoplasm of liver/intrahepatic bile ducts.

- *RCP report (1)* identifies opportunity to address 20 per cent of patient admissions to hospital for unrelated illnesses with potentially hazardous alcohol intake.

The main cause of cirrhosis in this country is excess alcohol consumption. Per capita consumption in the UK is increasing, whereas in mainland Europe it is showing a steady decrease. In fact, the UK, from low down in the league table of cirrhosis prevalence and mortality, has now reached the level of other European countries. Chronic liver disease from hepatitis B was considered to be rare in this country but the numbers infected have never been properly determined, and the Department of Health has estimated that an additional 6,000 new cases of chronic hepatitis B are coming into this country each year through legal immigration alone. Hepatitis C is much more frequent and of the estimated 400,000 cases in this country, only ten per cent have been diagnosed to date. The long natural history of this condition means that a substantial number of patients will not present with cirrhosis until in their 60s and 70s. Even if the infection has been recognised, the chances of having effective treatment in the UK are much smaller than in Europe generally. This is largely owing to the constraints effected by NICE in delaying consideration of the use of antiviral therapy. The newest form of interferon—Pegylated interferon, which has a much greater efficacy in terms of viral clearance and which has to be given only once instead of three times a week—being therefore much preferred by patients, will not be considered by NICE until later this year although it was licensed some time ago and elsewhere in Europe is being widely prescribed. Naturally, the Government wants to ensure that specialists on an expert network basis properly supervise such an expensive treatment, but it is very difficult to see how this can be implemented with the present lack of organisation of specialised services in hospitals, to which I will refer later.

Epidemiological studies are also showing an increase in the number of deaths from Hepatocellular cancer, which is not surprising as this tumour is a late complication of all types of cirrhosis. If the diagnosis can be made in the early stages when the tumour mass is small, treatment measures can be very effective in terms of prolongation of good quality life for several years. But early detection requires a much greater availability of ultrasound and CT machines as well as trained staff to run these machines. With the additional funding being pumped into the NHS at present, more machines are being installed, but there is a desperate shortage of radiographers and other support staff. What may become a new epidemic of cirrhosis, namely fatty liver disease is also giving rise to much concern. The disorder is related to obesity and diabetes, both of which are increasing in the UK as in other countries of the West. Perhaps ten per cent of these patients will finally progress to end-stage liver disease and with the long natural history of the condition the older age groups are likely to be particularly affected.

In hepatology, as with most other medical specialties, many more effective treatments are now available in comparison with 10-20 years ago, but virtually all require specialist knowledge and very often complex, hospital-based investigations. Most of the treatments, shown in Table 4:2 (p. 53), are limited in their use or 'rationed' to some extent in the UK by cost constraints, representing as they do new demands on the hospital's funds. Inevitably they will be more costly than the therapies—often ineffective—that were used before. Cost benefit analysis is now an integral part of the NICE considerations but until recently there have been almost constant deficits in hospital funding. Even if the new monies in the NHS were getting through to patient care, the greater expectations of patients as well as the cost of new remedies make it very difficult to see how the NHS, as currently funded and structured, can ever keep up. Of particular note amongst the list of treatments in Table 4:2, is vaccination against hepatitis B virus (HBV). Currently, we are one of the few remaining countries in Europe without universal vaccination of infants and children. The Department of Health decided HBV vaccination was not a cost effective procedure, a view that surely must change with the number of patients with this infection now being seen in this country.

Table 4:2
Lessening the impact of liver disease

Prevention	Lifestyle modification—alcohol, diet
	Universal HBV Vaccine
	Limited size packaging of Paracetamol
	Avoidance of herbal remedies
Antiviral Therapy	New agents for HBV (Lamivudine, Adefovir) and HCV (Pegylated Interferon)
Acute Liver Injury	Anti TNF, Pentoxifylline for alcoholic hepatitis
End Stage Disease	Liver support devices, Transplants (cadaver and living donor)
THE FUTURE	Genetic identification of disease susceptibility, reversal of liver damage by hepatocyte/stem cell implantation into liver

Direct and indirect rationing

With all the demands on primary care trusts for community care, it is difficult to see how agreement will ever be obtained for the shifting of funds toward specialty work and complex procedures even if funding is agreed for the common hospital services, such as hernias, other elective surgery, emergency medical admissions and so on. Within hospital trusts, the further distortions induced by Government initiatives are adding to the difficulties of setting priorities based on medical need. Furthermore, the lack of funds over the years coupled with the repeated reorganisation of the NHS have established an engrained culture of cannot do, rather than can do, in our hospitals.

Table 4:3
Rationing of care

DIRECT

1)   By NICE in delaying/not giving approval for new drugs, new devices

2)   By providers, i.e. Hospital Trusts and PCT's with conflicting priorities are limited (often deficient) funding

INDIRECT

1)   WL's for specialist investigations—CT's, Endoscopy, OP appointments, IP beds. Lack of personnel capacity within NHS and EU work hours directive

2)   Appropriated organisation for commissioning and funding of specialised services not yet in place

Indirect rationing, as shown in Table 4:3, covers all the limitations imposed by the shortage of equipment and, particularly, of staff. Waiting lists for consultant appointments and investigations remain too long in many areas, and there are often further delays in co-ordinating the doctor's opinions and results of investigations, let alone the patient's views regarding treatment. Most importantly, and often forgotten, are the limitations in care consequent on the failure to establish an organisational structure for the more specialised work to which I will return shortly.

This symposium is particularly concerned with the levels of care that the elderly may receive and my impression in hepatology is that, as in other specialties, they are generally restricted and that age limits are often imposed without any evidence base for them. Very little data is available in the UK, although the data from Europe is more encouraging. Figure 4:1 (p. 56), shows the number of liver transplants performed by age group since 1988, compared with earlier years. Certainly there are now a substantial number of patients in the 60-70 year age group who are receiving transplants, and in the over-70s age group, the number of cases is also increasing. Survival figures—again based on European Liver Transplant Registry data—for those aged 60 years plus are remarkably good and here the curves in Figure 4:2 (p. 57) extend up to ten years post-transplant. One would anticipate a requirement for a greater number of liver transplants in the older age groups consequent on the increased number of cases of cirrhosis in the UK already referred to and for whom transplantation may be the best option. The good results obtained reinforce the fact that elderly patients can have worthwhile benefit from therapies that are usually thought of as appropriate only to the younger age groups.

One limit to the wider use of transplantation is the falling number of cadaver livers becoming available because of a reduction in the number of road traffic accidents. Maximisation of organ retrieval rates requires government action in a number of areas but if certain measures were implemented, organ donation could be substantially increased as has been brought about in Spain. Another limit to transplantation in the UK is the small number of centres with recognition and funding for the procedure—six only—and which are not well distributed around the country. This is one factor, I believe, in why we in the UK have the lowest referral rate of end-stage liver disease patients for transplantation of all the European countries.

Figure 4:1
Age and sex distribution, May 1968 - December 2001

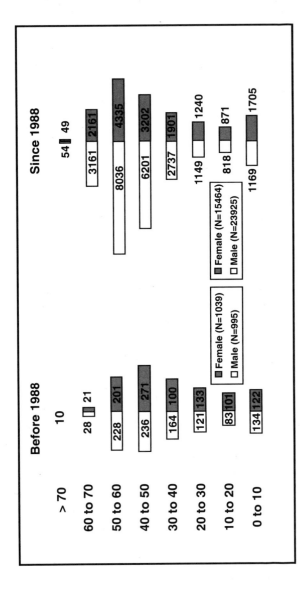

Source: European Liver Transplant Registry, 2002.

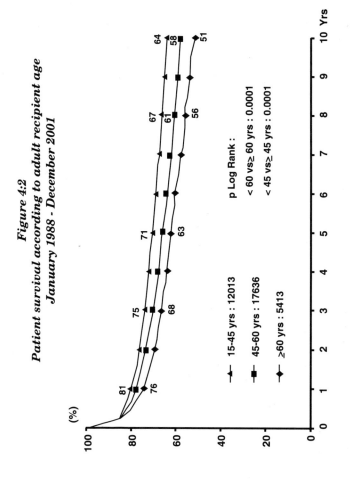

Figure 4:2
Patient survival according to adult recipient age
January 1988 - December 2001

(%)

p Log Rank :

< 60 vs ≥ 60 yrs : 0.0001

< 45 vs ≥ 45 yrs : 0.0001

15-45 yrs : 12013

45-60 yrs : 17636

≥60 yrs : 5413

10 Yrs

Source: European Liver Transplant Registry, 2002.

Commissioning of specialist services

In the UK, specialist services, almost all of which are hospital based, have since the early 1980s been separated into two categories. The supra-regional or national specialties represent a small number of highly complex medical or surgical treatments and investigations carried out in a restricted number of centres. These centres receive central (top-slice) funding based on an approved annual schedule of work and budget submission. Initially managed by an advisory group of the Department of Health, this was replaced in 1996, by the new government which set up a supposedly independent body known as National Specialist Commissioning Advisory Group (NSCAG). It was given a wider remit to cover guidelines and overall arrangements for a whole range of specialist work in addition to the supra-regional specialties.[2] Currently designated national services include liver transplants, cardio-thoracic transplants, certain congenital anomalies, severe personality disorders and so on. Indeed, the NSCAG controls a wide range of different specialties, 23 in all, representing a substantial amount of complex clinical work. Each large university hospital is likely to have one or two of such designated national services.

The largest category of specialist work in hospitals encompasses what has been termed the regional specialties on the basis of the geographical areas they serve and since some at least were initially developed with additional funding by the Regional Health Authorities in existence at that time (see Table 4:4, p. 59). Such services, which are normally provided in tertiary referral hospitals, relate to patients with complex or uncommon conditions, requiring a concentration of clinical care; a good example would be renal dialysis and renal transplants. Support for these specialties over the years has varied around the country according to different RHAs priorities and often also because of the failure to define what needed to be provided in its specialist centre rather than be distributed more widely over the region.

Table 4:4
Commissioning of regional specialities

1980s	Organisation and fundraising to variable extent by RHAs
1991	Responsibility given to DHAs with encouragement to set up consortia or lead HAs
1997	New Regional Specialised Commissioning Groups established (RSCGs)
1999	ECRs abolished
1999	Responsibility for commissioning and funding passed to PCTs - must work collaboratively, strategic HA to oversee
1999	RSCGs continued on temporary basis

In 1991, when the RHAs were abolished by the Conservative government, responsibility for the regional services was devolved to District Health Authorities, with encouragement to set up consortia or lead health authorities for the commissioning of such services. This was largely ignored and by 1996 a number of critical reports had appeared including those of CSAG and the Audit Commission. In 1997 with a new government and NHS white paper, specialist commissioning was given back to the regions with establishment of what were termed Regional Specialty Commissioning Groups (RSCGs). In 1999, the scheme of extra contractual referrals by which patients could be referred for tertiary care from smaller hospitals and which had largely been funding specialist work was abolished. The Government specifically did not allow the out-of-area payment scheme that replaced it to be used for specialist referrals, so cutting off funds needed for care and as a result greatly limiting the ability of patients with difficult clinical problems to be referred.

The new NHS plan in 2001 represented a major change— indeed a revolution!—with 75 per cent of the funding handed over to the primary care trusts (PCTs). The responsibility for specialist services was passed to them with the statement that they must work collaboratively and that the 28 new Strategic Health Authorities that replaced the District Health Authorities were to oversee it. RSCGs were continued on a temporary basis whilst the PCTs were being set up and in fact have done a considerable amount of work in what is known as the Specialist Services Definitions Set. This defines more precisely what is required of a specialist service in terms of expertise and facilities. By November 2001, as shown in Table 4:5 (p. 61), the definitions for 35 specialties had been drawn up and 23 of these have been published in the Department of Health website. However, relatively few consortia of PCTs had been set up for the commissioning and funding of such specialist services. I understand that for nine of them in the London RSCG, some form of consortia arrangement is now in place but that for only two or three of them are funds actually flowing through the lead PCT of the consortia to the provider services in the various hospital trust involved. The other seven RSCGs around the country have even fewer in place. The overall lack of progress was confirmed in a recent Hospital Doctor analysis of planning for specialist treatments obtained by the political consultancy Cicero.[3] This showed that out of a possible total of 208 points, nine of the 14 regions scored less than 50 and the highest score of the remainder was 71.5. The Academy of Medical Royal Colleges have also raised many concerns over the PCTs controlling the budgets and commissioning for specialised hospital services.[4]

I am sorry to say that Hepatology remains unrecognised and unfunded although a Definition Set No. 19 has been published, and currently efforts are being made to get consideration of this specialty into the work programme for the London RSCG next year, providing that the RSCGs remain in existence. Ministers commissioned a consultation paper on the RSCGs this year, which is due shortly. It is possible that we will end up with regional commissioning organised by RSCG or their successors, but based on funding from the PCTs and with binding agreements being placed on the transfer of funds—an arrangement that is likely to lead to maximum disagreement between the two parties.

Table 4:5
Regional specialised services definitions set

An outline specification for each speciality that could provide mechanism for accreditation and funding

- By November 2001—work on 35 specialities carried out with 23 published by DoH on web site

- By November 2002—within London RSCG, consortia set up for Bone Marrow TP (Set2), Haemophilia (Set 3), Spinal Services (4), Cleft Liver & Palate (15), Specialised Mental Health (22)—making nine in all

- The other seven RSCGs have one to two in place only

- Hepatology (Set 19) not yet included

Finally, I want to mention various current central government initiatives whose implementation will be very difficult without appropriate structures for specialist commissioning being first put in place. Thus in Hepatology, we have a Department of Health paper on developing services for hepatitis C patients. Many of the proposals are dependent on the presence of specialist centres looking after defined geographical areas and networks. Then there is the joint Cabinet Office/Department of Health group on the problems of alcoholism; the government, in the NHS plan, having committed itself to produce a national alcohol strategy by 2004. The effects of drinking on driving, anti-social behaviour and health issues ranging from accidents to serious clinical conditions are to be included in this strategy. The brief for the group refers to the 'joining up of government activity' but as I have repeatedly stressed we currently do not have the appropriate structures in place. Such a wide ranging alcohol strategy will also require links between the specialist liver centres and other structures/ bodies concerned with non-medical aspects of alcoholism.

Then there is the continuing work of NICE and the implementation of its recommendations. As shown in Figure 4:3 (below) there are no links between any of these initiatives and the central effecting body, namely the specialist liver unit. The latter's link with the PCTs (and therefore funding), is shown by a dotted line only reflecting the present state of uncertainty. The liver transplant centres stand separate in their funding and structure; and then there are National Cancer Networks, which include liver patients, and National Service Frameworks (NSFs), which set out a wider view of a national provision for quality care. There is no NSF planned for Liver Disease, but in the most recent NSF, that for Diabetes, the policy framework was published over a year ago and measures for implementation, which I understand are being drawn up by another body, are still awaited.

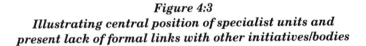

Figure 4:3
Illustrating central position of specialist units and present lack of formal links with other initiatives/bodies

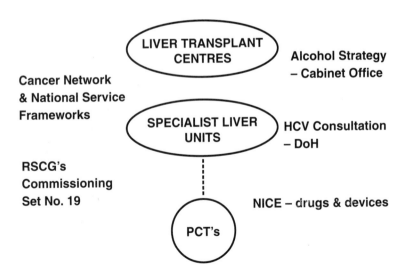

Table 4:6 summarises what I see as the most important issues relating to the proposed PCT commissioning and funding of specialised services. One wonders how long it will be before these are swept away by yet another reorganisation. The see-saw between local, regional and national provision over the years is surely an indictment of the direct involvement of governments in health care management. Rationing—directly and indirectly—is evident throughout the NHS, and relating to the subject of this symposium, the increasing number of elderly patients as well as the extent of current immigration, will all add to the unmet needs and demands on the service. Sadly to me, having been involved in specialist work since the 1960s, I see our place in the world league table on research and development falling steadily, and that other countries have been able to improve the standards of care far more than we have been able to do.

Table 4:6
***A summary and potential for success
in specialist commissioning***

Summary of main issues relating to PCT commissioning of specialised services

- Lack of coterminosity of specialist liver units (& networks) with PCTs consortia makes for administrative difficulties

- With the many priorities for PCTs in *local services*, loss of budget to specialist funding makes *for inevitable conflicts*

- Government initiatives for alcohol, HCV, Cancer Networks make for further difficulties with central specialist units commissioning not in place

- Restrictions on NSCAG funded units (23 specialties currently) and uncertain relationships to regional specialties not centrally funded (35 definitions set) distort clinical practice in specialty work

Notes

David G. Green and Benedict Irvine

1   OECD, *Health Data: A Comparative Analysis of 33 Countries*, Paris: OECD and CREDES, 2002.

2   Dobson, R., 'Proportion of spending on care for older people falls', *BMJ* 2002; 325:355 (17 August).

3   Seshamani, M. and Gray, A., 'The impact of ageing on expenditures in the National Health Service', *Age and Ageing,* Vol. 31, No. 4, 2002, pp. 287-94.

4   Grimley Evans, J., 'This patient or that patient', in Smith, R. (ed.), *Rationing in Action*, London: *BMJ*, 1993, p. 120. See also Grimley Evans, J., 'Rationing health care by age: the case against', *BMJ* 1997;314:822 (15 March).

5   Kee, F., *et al*, 'Urgency and priority for cardiac surgery: a clinical judgement analysis,' *BMJ* 1998;316:925-929 (21 March).

6   Jee, M. and Or, Z., *Health Outcomes in OECD Countries: A Framework of Health Indicators for Outcome-Orientated Policy Making*, Labour market and social policy – Occasional Papers, No. 36, Paris: OECD, 1999, p. 63. Rates of immunisations, of preventive screening for blood pressure, cholesterol and cancers, the percentage of pregnant women receiving prenatal care in the first trimester, and so forth are other potential indicators of effective healthcare interventions.

7   OECD ARD team, 'Summary of Results from Ischaemic Heart Disease Study', *What is Best and at What Cost? OECD Study on Cross-National Differences of Ageing Related Diseases*, OECD Working Party on Social Policy, Ageing-Related Diseases, Concluding Workshop, Paris, 20-21 June 2002, pp. 13-16.

8   MacLeod, M.C.M. *et al*, 'Geographic, demographic, and socioeconomic variations in the investigation and management of coronary heart disease in Scotland', *Heart* 1999;81:252-56.

9   MacLeod, *et al*, 1998.

10 Bufalari, A., *et al*, 'Surgical care in octogenarians', *British Journal of Surgery*, 1996, Vol. 83, pp. 1783-87.

11 OECD, ARD team, 'Summary of Stroke Disease Study' (Draft), *What is Best and at What Cost? OECD Study on Cross-National Differences of Ageing Related Diseases*, DEELSA/ELSWP1/ARD(2002)4. OECD Working Party on Social Policy, Ageing-Related Diseases, Concluding Workshop, Paris, 20-21 June 2002.

12 Sutton, G., 'Will you still need me, will you still screen me, when I'm past 64?', *BMJ* 1997;315:1032-33 (25 October).

13 Sutton, 1997.

14 van Dijck, J.A. *et al*, 'Mammographic screening after the age of 65 years: evidence for a reduction in breast cancer mortality,' *International Journal of Cancer* 1996; 66:727-731.

15 OECD ARD team, 'Summary of Results from Breast Cancer Disease Study', *What is Best and at What Cost? OECD Study on Cross-National Differences of Ageing Related Diseases*, OECD Working Party on Social Policy, Ageing-Related Diseases, Concluding Workshop, Paris, 20-21 June 2002, p. 9.

16 DoH, *Building on Experience, Breast Screening Programme Annual Review 2002,* NHS, 2002. The Annual Report (2003) of the NHS Modernisation Board acknowledges that this reform is underway; roughly 100,000 more women were invited to be screened in the year to October 2002 (The Annual Report (2003) of the NHS Modernisation Board).

17 Morrison, A.S. *et al*, 'Breast cancer incidence and mortality in the Breast Cancer Detection Demonstration Project,' *Journal of the National Cancer Institute*, Vol. 80, No. 19, 7 December 1998, pp. 1540-47.

18 Quinn, M.J., Martinez-Garcia, C., Berrino, F. and the EUROCARE Working Group, 'Variation in survival from breast cancer in Europe by age and country, 1978-1989', *European Journal of Cancer*, Vol. 14, No. 14, 1998, pp. 2204-11.

19 OECD ARD team, 'Summary of Results from Breast Cancer Disease Study', 2002, p. 21.

20 OECD ARD team, 'Summary of Results from Breast Cancer Disease Study', 2002.

21 OECD ARD team, 'Summary of Results from Breast Cancer Disease Study', 2002, pp. 4-7.

22 OECD ARD team, 'Summary of Results from Breast Cancer Disease Study', 2002, p. 18.

23 OECD ARD team, 'Summary of Results from Breast Cancer Disease Study', 2002, pp. 18-19.

24 OECD ARD team, 'Summary of Results from Breast Cancer Disease Study', 2002, p. 20.

25 Turner, N.J., 'Cancer in old age—is it inadequately investigated and treated?', *BMJ* 1999; 319:309-312 (31 July).

26 *OECD Health Data: A Comparative Analysis of 33 Countries*, Paris: OECD and CREDES, 2002. French figure relates to 1999.

Stephen Pollard

1 Burt, C., 'National trends in the use of medications in office-based practice, 1985-1999', *Health Affairs*, 21(4), 206-214, July/August 2002.

2 United Nations, *World population aging: 1950-2050*, New York: United Nations, 2002.

3 Federal Interagency Forum on Aging-Related Statistics, 2002; Freedman, 2002, 2000, 1998. Federal Interagency Forum on Aging-Related Statistics. Older Americans 2000: key indicators of well-being. Federal Interagency Forum on Aging-Related Statistics. Washington, DC: US Government Printing Office, 2000; Freedman, V.A., Aykan, H. and Martin, L.G., 'Another look at aggregate changes in severe cognitive impairment', *Journal of Gerontology*, Series B, Psychological Sciences and Social Sciences, 56(2), S100-11, 2002; Freedman, V.A., Martin, L.G., 'Contribution of chronic conditions to aggregate changes in old-age functioning', *American Journal of Public Health* 90(11), 1755-60, 2000; Freedman, V.A. and Martin, L.G., 'Understanding trends in functional limitations among older Americans', *American Journal of Public Health* 88(10), 1457-62, 1998.

4   Vital Statistics Data, National Center for Health Statistics.

5   US Department of Health and Human Services report, 'Securing the Benefits of Medical Innovation for Seniors: The Role of Prescription Drugs and Drug Coverage'.

6   LDL-cholesterol—Low density lipoproteins; often referred to as 'bad cholesterol'.

John Grimley Evans

1   Jones, H.B., 'The relation of human health to age, place, and time' in Birren, J.E. (ed.), *Handbook of Aging and the Individual*, Chicago: University of Chicago Press, 1959, pp. 336-63.

2   Grimley Evans, J., 'A correct compassion. The medical response to an ageing society', *J Roy Coll Phys* (Lond) 31, 674-684, 1997.

3   Martin, J., Meltzer, H. and Elliot, D., 'The prevalence of disability among adults', *OPCS Surveys of Disability in Great Britain: Report 1*, Office of Population Censuses and Surveys Social Survey Division, London: Her Majesty's Stationery Office, 1988.

4   Eatwell, J. (1999). 'The anatomy of the pensions "crisis"', in *Economic survey of Europe*, No. 3, Economic Commission for Europe, ed., Geneva: United Nations, 1999, pp. 57-61.

5   Zweifel, P., Felder, S. and Meiers, M. (1999) 'Ageing of population and health care expenditure: A red herring?', *Health Economics*, 8 (6), pp.485-496.

6   Grimley Evans, J., 'Evidence-based and evidence-biased medicine', *Age Ageing*, 24, 1995, pp. 461-63.

7   Manton, K.G. and Gu, X., 'Changes in the prevalence of chronic disability in the United States black and nonblack population above age 65 from 1982 to 1999', *Proceedings of the National Academy of Sciences*, USA, 2001; 98(11): 6454-6359.

8   The Norwegian Multicenter Study Group, 'Timolol-induced reduction in mortality and reinfarction in patients surviving acute myocardial infarction', *New England J Med* 1981; 304(14):801-807.

9 Grimley Evans, J., 'Prevention of age-associated loss of autonomy: epidemiological approaches', *J Chron Dis* 37:353-363, 1984.

10 The Carnegie Inquiry into the Third Age, Final Report: Life, work and livelihood in the third age, Dunfermline: The Carnegie United Kingdom Trust, 1993.

Roger Williams

1 'Royal College of Physicians Report on Alcohol - Can the NHS Afford it? Recommendations for a coherent alcohol strategy for hospitals', published by the Working Party of the RCP, February 2001.

2 National Specialist Commissioning Advisory Group Annual Report, 2001 - 2001, Department of Health Website.

3 'Will hospitals cope with swing in buying-power?', *Hospital Doctor*, feature 23, 21 November, 2002.

4 'Academy of Medical Royal Colleges Report Specialist Services: Is the future secure?', Academy of Medical Royal Colleges Website.

Glossary

Bisphosphonates
Including, for example, alendronate and risedronate), first introduced in the mid-1990s, and which inhibit bone reabsorption, are one recent category of pharmaceuticals that effectively treat osteoporosis.

Bone reabsorption
Process occurring throughout life, by which old bone is removed by cells called osteoclasts. Old bone is then replaced by new bone.

Cytotoxic drugs
Cytotoxic drugs are used to combat cancer. They fall naturally into a number of classes, each with characteristic anti-tumour activity, sites of action, and toxicity.

Genomics
The study of genes and their function.

Gleevec
Gleevec, which is used to treat chronic myeloid leukemia (CML), is one of the first agents using this new approach that targets abnormal proteins fundamental to the cancer. Unlike most current cancer therapies that kill both normal and cancer cells leading to unwanted side-effects, Gleevec and other drugs in this class are designed to zero in on specific cancer-causing molecules, eliminating cancer cells while avoiding serious damage to other, non-cancerous cells. Early studies of this drug have shown that in patients with chronic myelocytic leukemia, white blood-cell counts are restored to normal levels.

Ischaemic
Caused by inadequate supply of blood to an organ.

LDL-cholesterol
Low density lipoproteins; often referred to as 'bad cholesterol'.

69

Proteomics	The study of proteins and their functions.
NICE	National Institute for Clinical Excellence. In the UK NICE assesses therapies and provides guidelines for their use.
SSRIs	Selective serotonin reuptake inhibitors are used to treat depression and have significantly fewer side effects than older drugs, making it easier for patients, including older adults, to adhere to treatment.
Thrombolytic agent	Known as a 'clot-busting' drugs, thrombolytic agents such as Tissue Plasminogen Activator (t-PA), can dissolve the blood clots that cause most heart attacks and strokes.

Independence: The Institute for the Study of Civil Society (CIVITAS) is a registered educational charity (No. 1085494) and a company limited by guarantee (No. 04023541). CIVITAS is financed from a variety of private sources to avoid over-reliance on any single or small group of donors.

All publications are independently refereed. All the Institute's publications seek to further its objective of promoting the advancement of learning. The views expressed are those of the authors, not of the Institute.